Mawaddah Azman
Siti Zulaili Zulkepli
Abdullah Sani Mohamed

Insulin Resistance using HOMA model in Obstructive Sleep Apnea

Mawaddah Azman
Siti Zulaili Zulkepli
Abdullah Sani Mohamed

Insulin Resistance using HOMA model in Obstructive Sleep Apnea

LAP LAMBERT Academic Publishing

Impressum / Imprint
Bibliografische Information der Deutschen Nationalbibliothek: Die Deutsche Nationalbibliothek verzeichnet diese Publikation in der Deutschen Nationalbibliografie; detaillierte bibliografische Daten sind im Internet über http://dnb.d-nb.de abrufbar.

Alle in diesem Buch genannten Marken und Produktnamen unterliegen warenzeichen-, marken- oder patentrechtlichem Schutz bzw. sind Warenzeichen oder eingetragene Warenzeichen der jeweiligen Inhaber. Die Wiedergabe von Marken, Produktnamen, Gebrauchsnamen, Handelsnamen, Warenbezeichnungen u.s.w. in diesem Werk berechtigt auch ohne besondere Kennzeichnung nicht zu der Annahme, dass solche Namen im Sinne der Warenzeichen- und Markenschutzgesetzgebung als frei zu betrachten wären und daher von jedermann benutzt werden dürften.

Bibliographic information published by the Deutsche Nationalbibliothek: The Deutsche Nationalbibliothek lists this publication in the Deutsche Nationalbibliografie; detailed bibliographic data are available in the Internet at http://dnb.d-nb.de.

Any brand names and product names mentioned in this book are subject to trademark, brand or patent protection and are trademarks or registered trademarks of their respective holders. The use of brand names, product names, common names, trade names, product descriptions etc. even without a particular marking in this work is in no way to be construed to mean that such names may be regarded as unrestricted in respect of trademark and brand protection legislation and could thus be used by anyone.

Coverbild / Cover image: www.ingimage.com

Verlag / Publisher:
LAP LAMBERT Academic Publishing
ist ein Imprint der / is a trademark of
OmniScriptum GmbH & Co. KG
Heinrich-Böcking-Str. 6-8, 66121 Saarbrücken, Deutschland / Germany
Email: info@lap-publishing.com

Herstellung: siehe letzte Seite /
Printed at: see last page
ISBN: 978-3-659-76336-6

Zugl. / Approved by: Kuala Lumpur, Universiti Kebangsaan Malaysia, Dissertation submitted in partial fulfillment of the Degree of Master of Surgery in Otorhinolaryngology, Head and Neck, 2013

Copyright © 2015 OmniScriptum GmbH & Co. KG
Alle Rechte vorbehalten. / All rights reserved. Saarbrücken 2015

Authors

Corresponding author:

Dr. Mawaddah Azman
MS (ORL, Head and Neck Surgery-UKM)
Department of Otorhinolaryngology, 9th floor, Clinical Block, Hospital Universiti Kebangsaan Malaysia, Jalan Yaakob Latiff, 54100 Bandar Tun Razak, Cheras, Kuala Lumpur, Malaysia.
Tel: +60391455555, +60163061959
E mail: mawaddah1504@yahoo.com

Role:

Substantial contributions in acquisition, analysis, or interpretation of data for the work; AND Drafting the work or revising it critically for important intellectual content; AND Final approval of the version to be published; AND Agreement to be accountable for all aspects of the work in ensuring that questions related to the accuracy or integrity of any part of the work are appropriately investigated and resolved.

Author(s):

Dr. Siti Zulaili Zulkepli,
MS (ORL, Head and Neck Surgery-UKM)
Department of Otorhinolaryngology,
Hospital Angkatan Tentera,
Kem Terendak,
Melaka.

Role:

Substantial contributions in acquisition, analysis, or interpretation of data for the work; AND Final approval of the version to be published;

Clinical Professor Dato' Dr. Abdullah Sani,
FRCS (Edin), MS (ORL, Head and Neck Surgery-UKM),
Department of Otorhinolaryngology,
Lecturer and Senior Consultant,
Universiti Kebangsaan Malaysia,
Kuala Lumpur.

Role :

Substantial contributions in conceptualization for the work; AND Final approval of the version to be published; AND Agreement to be accountable for all aspects of the work in ensuring that questions related to the accuracy or integrity of any part of the work are appropriately investigated and resolved.

CONTENTS

	PAGE
CONTENTS	3
LIST OF FIGURES	4
LIST OF TABLES	5
ABSTRACT	6
CHAPTER 1: INTRODUCTION	7
CHAPTER 2: MATERIALS AND METHODS	11
CHAPTER 3: RESULTS	15
CHAPTER 4: DISCUSSION	32
CHAPTER 5: CONCLUSION	37
REFERENCES	39
APPENDIX	45
ACKNOWLEDGEMENT	51

LIST OF FIGURES

	PAGE
Figure 1: Study flow	14
Figure 2: Gender distribution	16
Figure 3: Race distribution	17
Figure 4: Age distribution	18
Figure 5: Distribution of patients according to OSA severity and insulin resistance	19
Figure 6: Correlation between AHI and HOMA IR	21
Figure 7: Distribution of patients according to ESS category and insulin resistance	22
Figure 8: Correlation between ESS and HOMA IR	24
Figure 9: Distribution of patients according to BMI category and insulin resistance	25
Figure 10: Correlation between BMI and HOMA IR	27
Figure 11: Correlation between waist circumference and HOMA IR	29

LIST OF TABLES

	PAGE
Table 1: Inclusion and Exclusion Criteria	12
Table 2: Comparison of mean HOMA IR with AHI group	20
Table 3: Comparison of mean HOMA IR with ESS score	23
Table 4: Comparison of mean HOMA IR with BMI categories	26
Table 5: Comparison of HOMA IR and mean of Waist Circumference	28
Table 6: Distribution of patients across OSA parameters and HOMA IR values	31

ABSTRACT

Introduction: Obstructive sleep apnea (OSA) is a common disease and is associated with significant cardiovascular, cerebrovascular, and metabolic complications. Current evidences show inconclusive association between OSA and insulin resistance (IR). This study aims to examine possible correlation between OSA parameters and IR. **Design:** This was a cross-sectional study to examine the association between OSA parameters and IR using homeostasis model assessment (HOMA) on patients who underwent polysomnogram (PSG) in a tertiary center between March 2011 and March 2012 (1 year). **Materials and Methods:** A total of 62 patients underwent PSG within the study period, of which 16 patients were excluded due to abnormal fasting blood sugar. Information on patients' medical illnesses, medications, and Epworth sleepiness scale (ESS) was obtained. Patients' body mass index (BMI), neck circumference, and waist circumference (WC) were measured. Blood samples were collected after 8 hours of fasting to measure HOMA–IR value. Overnight PSG was performed for all patients. Data was recorded and analyzed using SPSS, version 12.0 (SPSS Inc, Chicago, USA). **Results:** The prevalence of IR in OSA patients was 64.3%. There was significant correlation between OSA parameters (apnea-hypopnea index, ESS, BMI, and WC) and HOMA–IR with correlation coefficient of 0.529, 0.224, 0.261, and 0.354, respectively. **Conclusion:** A linear correlation exists between OSA parameters and IR concluding a definite causal link between OSA and IR. IR screening is recommended in severe OSA patients.

CHAPTER 1

INTRODUCTION

Obstructive sleep apnea (OSA) is a condition characterized by recurrent complete or partial upper airway obstructions during sleep with each episode generally being terminated by arousal when upper airway muscle tone increases[1]. Clinical symptoms of OSA include loud snoring, witnessed breathing pauses by a bed-partner, choking or gasping during sleep, morning headache, and daytime sleepiness[2]. Obstructive sleep apnea however can be present without significant symptomatology[2]. When OSA is accompanied by symptoms, most commonly excessive daytime sleepiness, it has been labeled as the OSA syndrome (OSAS)[2].

Obstructive apnea is defined as cessation of airflow due to upper airway collapse lasting at least 10 seconds. Obstructive hypopneas are characterized by either a ≥50% decrease in airflow from baseline lasting at least 10 seconds associated with a 4% oxygen desaturation[3]. The standard diagnostic test for OSA is an overnight polysomnogram (PSG) which consists of continuous polygraph recording from surface leads for electroencephalography, electrooculography, electromyography, electrocardiography, thermistors for nasal and oral airflow, thoracic and abdominal impedance belts for respiratory effort, pulse oximeter for oxyhemoglobin level, tracheal microphone for snoring, and sensors for leg and sleep position[4]. Information from the PSG is reported as the apnea hypopnea index (AHI), used to categorize the severity of OSA and it represents the average number of apneas and/or hypopneas per hour of recorded sleep. In adults, an AHI less than 5 events per hour is considered normal. Mild OSA is defined as an AHI between 5 and 15 events per hour, moderate OSA between 16 and 30 events per hour and severe OSA as greater than 30 events per hour[3]. The prevalence of OSA in middle-aged adults between 30 and 60 years of age has been reported as 9% for women and 24% for men[5].

OSA is associated with increased cardiovascular and cerebrovascular morbidity [6]. It is also recognized that many subjects with OSA have central obesity[7] and other features of metabolic syndrome[8,9], namely hyperinsulinemia, glucose intolerance, insulin resistance, dyslipidemia and hypertension[10]. These features of the metabolic syndrome are also known as the 'insulin resistance syndrome'[10].

Insulin resistance refers to a reduction in the expected physiologic action of insulin due to desensitization of peripheral tissue to insulin[10]. Increased insulin resistance is a primary characteristic of type 2 diabetes mellitus as well as an independent risk factor for hypertension and coronary heart disease[11]. Insulin resistance is said to be frequently observed in pre diabetic states. Type 2 Diabetes Mellitus will later develop when normoglycemia is no longer maintained as a result of inadequate pancreatic β cell compensation and insulin production[12]. Various methods have been developed to evaluate insulin resistance including hyperinsulinemic euglycemic clamp, the insulin suppression test and the frequently sampled intravenous glucose tolerance test. These tests however are expensive and have limited patient acceptance for use in large-scale studies[13].

The homeostasis model assessment (HOMA) has been proposed to assess secretion and resistance using the fasting glucose and insulin concentration and provides a good correlation for insulin resistance[13,14]. The formula for the HOMA model is given below:

$$\text{HOMA IR} = \frac{\text{Fasting insulin (µU/ml)} \times \text{Fasting glucose (mmol/L)}}{22.5}$$

By the formulation, HOMA IR value of more than three (3) defines patients with insulin resistance [15].

There are different hypotheses concerning the relationship between OSA and increased insulin resistance. The proposed mechanism is activation of a stress response by hypoxia and hypercapnia which occur during each apneic episodes in sleep. This stress response will in turn trigger the release of catecholamine and cortisol that lead to insulin resistance[16].

The possibility of a causal link is based on the observation from several studies that sleep loss and hypoxemia are independently associated with glucose intolerance and insulin resistance[17-21]. More recent clinic based studies found that patients with sleep-disordered breathing have significantly higher fasting glucose and insulin level compared with a group of weight-matched control subjects [22-24].

While there is no local data on incidence of OSA with insulin resistance in Malaysia as yet, we wish to test the hypothesis that OSA is an independent risk for insulin resistance. We would also want to see its correlation on disease severity by comparing with OSA-related parameters. Positive results and information from this study can be used in future for the need of insulin resistance screening in OSA patients. Funding for this study was provided by Universiti Kebangsaan Malaysia (UKM) Fundamental Research Grant and the conduct of this study was approved by UKM Medical Center Ethical Review Board in March 2011.

CHAPTER 2

MATERIALS AND METHOD

This was a cross sectional study whereby all patients undergoing polysomnogram (PSG) test in UKM Medical Center were recruited. Patients were recruited by convenient sampling from March 2011 until March 2012. The sample comprised of patients aged 20-60 years, mainly males (79%) and from Malay race (71.4%). This research project was approved by the UKM Medical Center Ethical Review Board and written informed consent was obtained. All procedures contributing to this work comply with the ethical standards of the relevant national and institutional guidelines and with the Helsinki Declaration of 1975, as revised in 2008.

Patients with factors which could affect insulin resistance were excluded, such as current substance use, having any endocrine disorder other than diabetes mellitus or insulin/steroidal pharmacotherapy (Table 1).

Table 1: Inclusion and Exclusion Criteria

Inclusion Criteria
• Adult patients between 18 and 65 years of age
• Patients whom consented and agreed for PSG and blood taking.
Exclusion Criteria
• Patient with known diabetes mellitus on medication.
• Patient with undiagnosed diabetes mellitus with fasting blood sugar of more than 7.0mmol/L.
• Patient with acromegaly.
• Patient with chronic renal failure.
• Patient with chronic liver disease
• Patient on systemic steroid treatment.
• Patient with Cushing's Syndrome
• Patient with thyroid disorder
• Patient on Thiazide or Thiazide-like diuretics
• Patient on Beta Blocker
• Patient on hormonal replacement therapy.
• Pregnancy.

Information on patient's baseline characteristics, illness(es), medication(s) and Epworth Sleepiness Scale (ESS) was sought from the patient, caregiver (where available) and patient's notes. Patient's weight, height, neck and waist circumference were measured. Neck circumference was taken at the level laryngeal prominence and waist circumference at the level of midpoint in between 12th rib and iliac crest. Blood samples were taken after at least eight hours of fasting. Two mls of blood was collected in fluoride oxalate bottle to be processed via chemistry method using Cobas Integra 700 (Roche Diagnostics) to yield fasting plasma glucose (mmol/L). For fasting serum insulin (µIU/ml), 3 mls of blood was collected in a plain tube, centrifuged at 3000 rpm for 10 minutes and frozen at −20 degrees Celsius. The samples were processed via chemiluminescent method using Immulite 2000 Immunoassay Analyzer system (Siemens Medical Solutions Diagnostic). The intra-assay coefficient of variation was 5.2- 6.4% while the interassay coefficient of variation was 5.9-8%.

All PSG were performed in an isolated room, using a computer-assisted sleep study device (SOMNOCheck Effort Weinmann, Hamburg, Germany). Parameters include AHI, apneas, hypopneas, arousal index, respiratory disturbance index and minimum oxygen saturation were documented.

Data analysis was done using the Statistical Package for Social Studies (SPSS) Version 12.0. Continuous data such as age, body mass index (BMI), neck and waist circumference and ESS score was tested for association with HOMA-IR. Comparisons of continuous clinical parameter between subjects with different categorization were made by ANOVA test and for a difference in mean of independent categories involved, were compared by t-tests. Pearson correlation was used to examine the association of two parameters.

Figure 1: Study flow

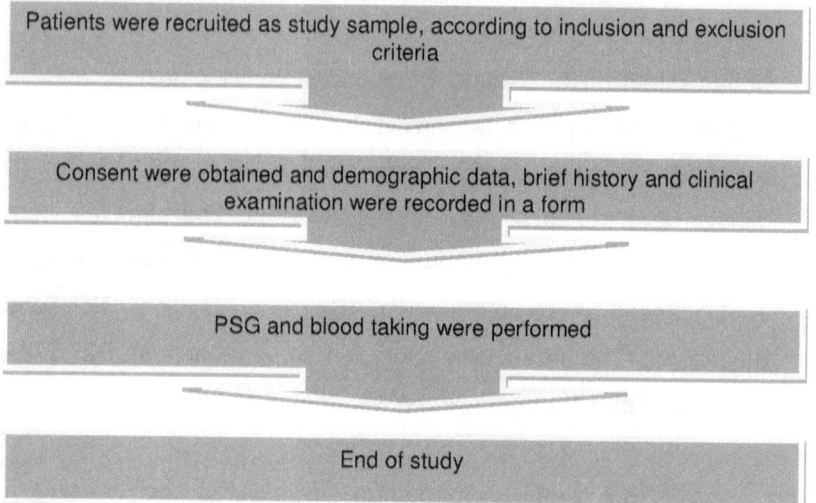

CHAPTER 3

RESULTS

From March 2011 until March 2012, 62 patients were referred to Otorhinolaryngology clinic UKM Medical Center for suspected sleep apnea and underwent polysomnogram (PSG) test but only 46 patients were recruited. Four patients refused to participate and another 12 patients were excluded because they were known to have Diabetes Mellitus.

All 46 patients underwent PSG followed by blood taking for fasting plasma glucose and fasting serum insulin within a week period of PSG date. Following blood investigations, another four patients were excluded as they were newly diagnosed Diabetes Mellitus with fasting blood sugar level of more than 7.0mmol/L. This is in keeping with our exclusion criteria. Thus the final number of patients that were studied was 42.

3.1 DEMOGRAPHIC DATA

3.1.1 Gender

42 patients were recruited for this study. 33 patients (79%) were males and nine patients (21%)were females. This is illustrated in Figure 2.

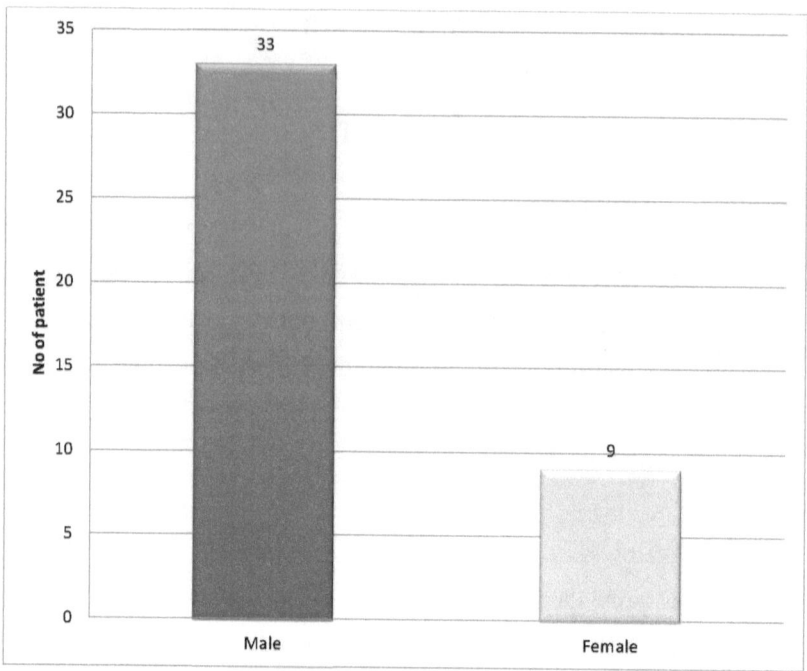

Figure 2: Gender distribution

3.1.2 Race

The majority of our study samples were from Malay population. They were 30 patients in number (71.4%). Chinese patients were eight and Indians were four in number.

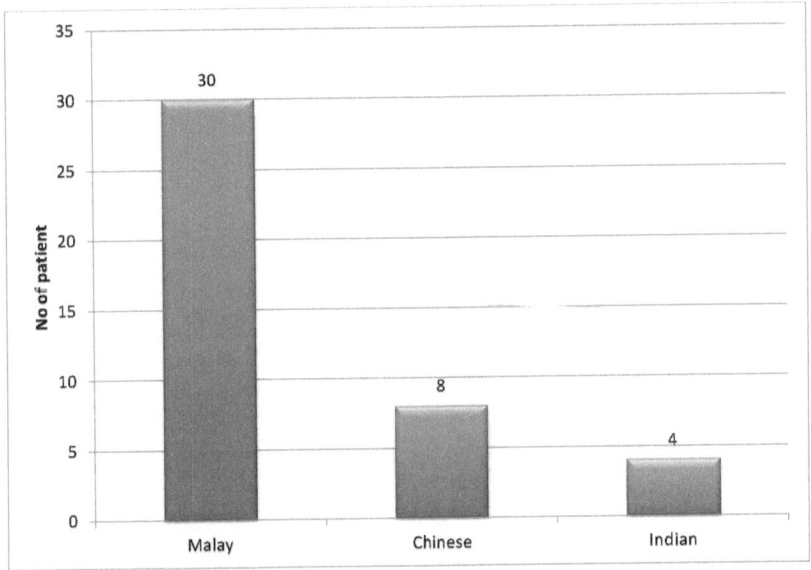

Figure 3: Race distribution

3.1.3 Age

In our study, the youngest patient was at 20 years of age while the eldest was 60 years old. Mean age of patients was 36.52 ± 8.93. Patients in the age range 30 to 39 years old makes up the majority 47.6% in this study as illustrated in Figure 4.

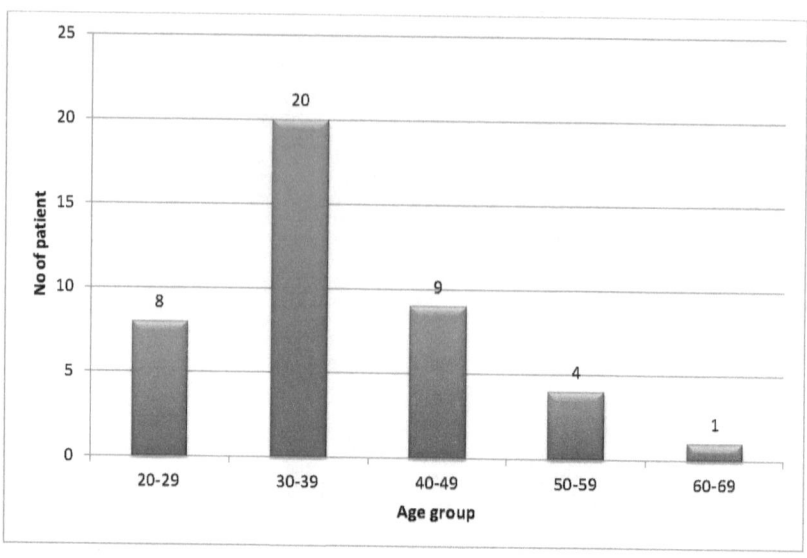

Figure 4: Age distribution

3.2 AHI AND INSULIN RESISTANCE

From a total of 42 patients that were included in this study, 28 patients (66.7%) were diagnosed to have OSA of varying degrees; majority in severe group (40.5%). Out of the 28 patients, 18 patients had significant HOMA IR value of more than three. The prevalence of insulin resistance amongst OSA patients in this study population is 64.3%.

The distribution of patients according to OSA severity and HOMA IR value is illustrated in Figure 5. Majority of patients with HOMA IR value of more than 3, which is significant for insulin resistance were in the severe OSA group. While those in mild and moderate OSA categories were two and one patient respectively.

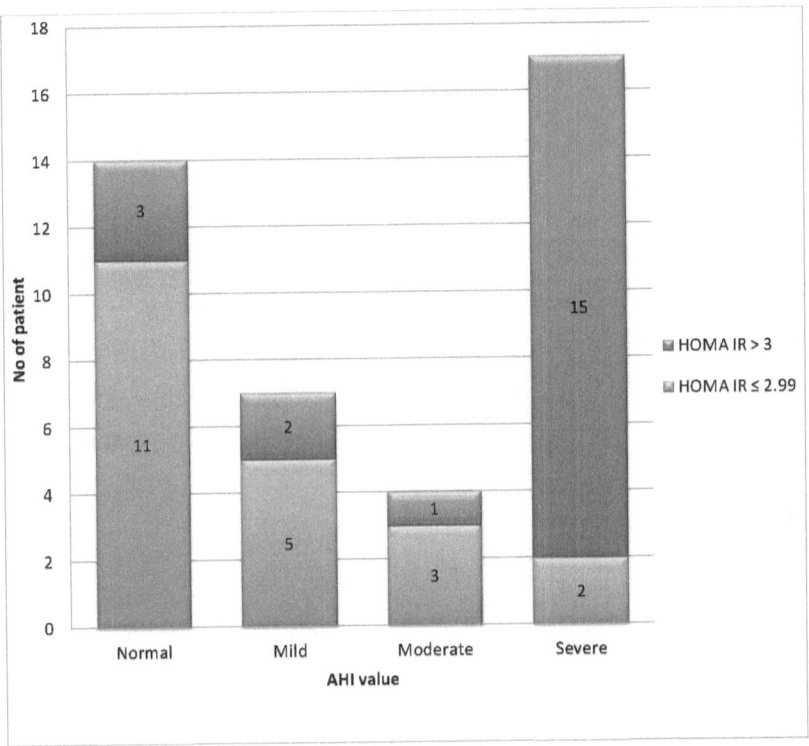

Figure 5: Distribution of patients according to OSA severity and insulin resistance

Comparisons were made between mean of HOMA IR value with severity of OSA using the ANOVA test. Statistical analysis revealed significant difference of mean HOMA IR between AHI groups with p value of 0.001 ($p<0.05$) (Table 2).

Table 2: Comparison of mean HOMA IR with AHI group

AHI	N	Mean HOMA IR
Normal	14	1.99± 1.49
Mild	7	2.12± 1.21
Moderate	4	1.83 ± 1.06
Severe	17	4.16± 1.41

p=0.001

Further correlation study was done using 2-tailed Pearson Correlation analysis. The study revealed significant correlation between HOMA IR and AHI (r=0.72 p<0.05). Further analysis from scatter plot regression is illustrated by Figure 6, which showed a high significant correlation between HOMA IR and AHI (R^2 = 0.529).

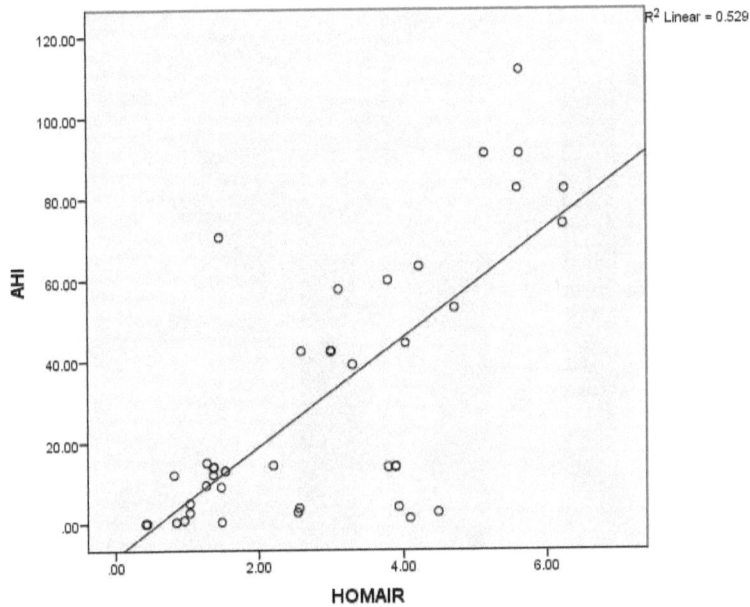

Figure 6: Correlation between AHI and HOMA IR

3.3 ESS AND INSULIN RESISTANCE

Mean ESS in this study is 11.36 ± 4.89. The lowest and highest score was 3 and 22 respectively. 17 patients (40.5%) scored their level of daytime sleepiness in normal category. While 22 other patients were equally distributed in mild and moderate groups. Three (7.1%) others scored their symptoms as severe. All of patients in severe ESS group had HOMA IR value of more than three. This is illustrated in Figure 7.

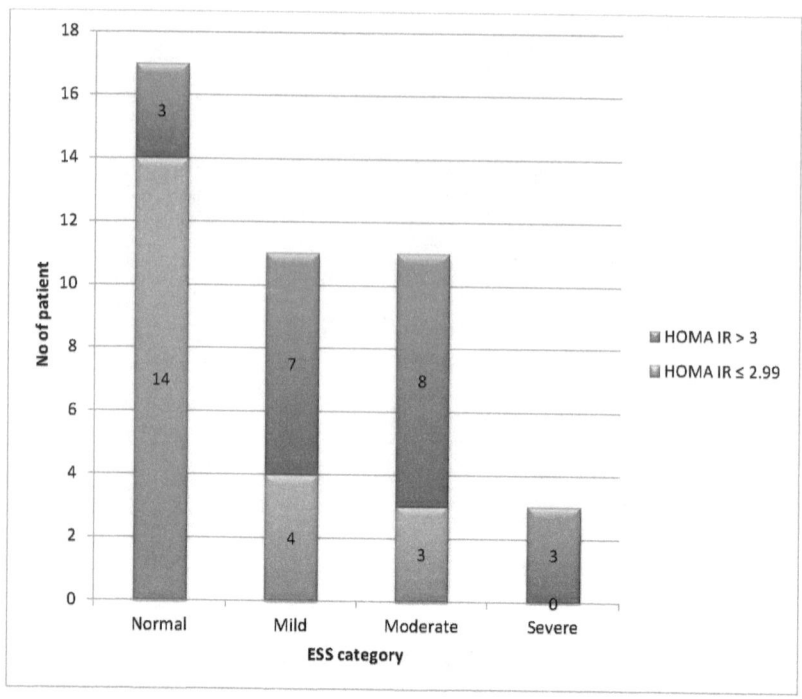

Figure 7: Distribution of patients according to ESS category and insulin resistance

Comparison of ESS score and HOMA IR value was assessed using the ANOVA test (Table 3). Statistical analysis revealed significant difference of mean HOMA IR between ESS score with p value equal to 0.01 ($p<0.05$).

Table 3: Comparison of mean HOMA IR with ESS score

ESS	N	Mean HOMA IR
Normal	17	1.90± 1.30
Mild	11	3.11± 1.66
Moderate	11	3.59 ± 1.63
Severe	3	4.74± 1.50

p=0.01

Correlation between ESS and insulin resistance was assessed using 2-tailed Pearson Correlation analysis. The study revealed significant correlation between HOMA IR and ESS score (r=0.47 p<0.05). Further analysis from scatter plot regression is illustrated in Figure 8, which showed significant correlation between HOMA IR and ESS score ($R^2 = 0.224$).

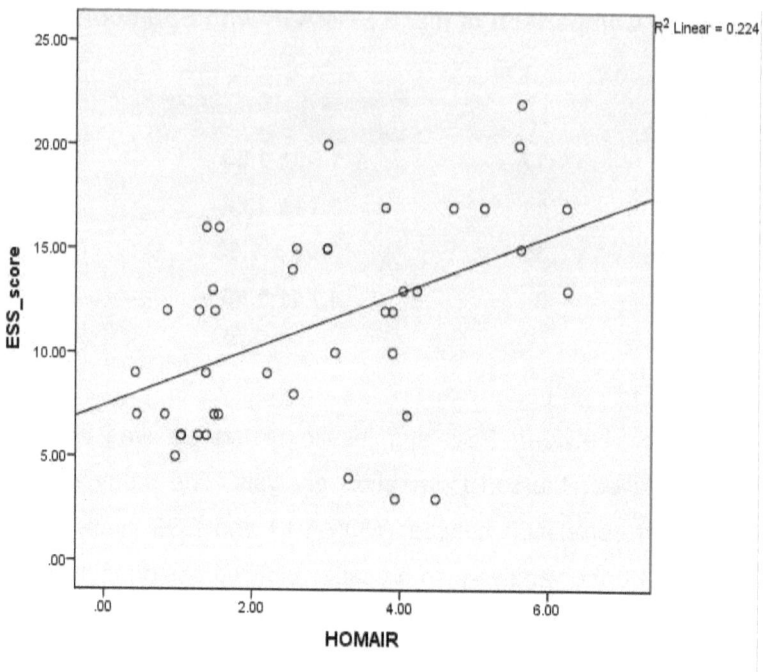

Figure 8: Correlation between ESS and HOMA IR

3.4 BMI AND INSULIN RESISTANCE

The BMI distribution of the study population was normal with mean value of 31.50 ± 6.89. Majority are categorized in obese 1 group (47.6%) at 27.5 to less than 35 kg/m².

Figure 9 below illustrated the distribution of patients according to BMI category and HOMA IR value. Patients in the obese 2 category (35 to < 40 kg/m^2) had highest percentage of insulin resistance (83.3%) followed by those in obese 3 category (60%).

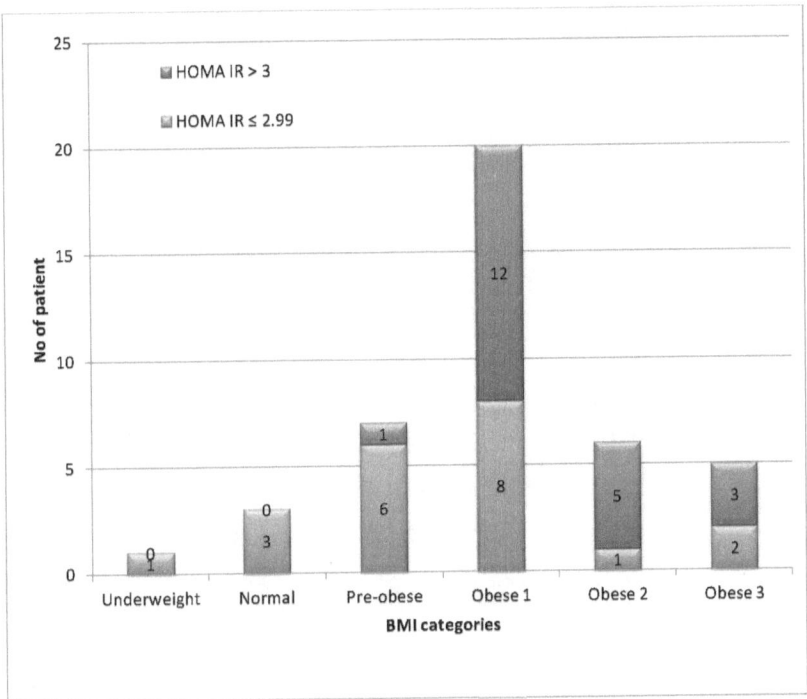

Figure 9 Distribution of patients according to BMI category and insulin resistance

Comparison of mean for each categorical BMI with HOMA IR value was also assessed using the ANOVA test. Statistical analysis revealed significant difference of mean HOMA IR and BMI groups with p value equal to 0.01 (p<0.05).

Table 4: Comparison of mean HOMA IR with BMI categories

BMI	N	Mean HOMA IR
Underweight	1	1.28
Normal	3	1.16± 0.28
Preobese	7	1.29 ± 0.72
Obese 1	20	3.19± 1.48
Obese 2	6	3.65± 1.74
Obese 3	5	4.17± 1.97

p=0.01

Correlation between BMI and insulin resistance was assessed using 2-tailed Pearson Correlation analysis. The study revealed significant correlation between HOMA IR and BMI (r=0.51 p<0.05). Further analysis from scatter plot regression is illustrated in Figure 10, which showed significant correlation between HOMA IR and BMI (R^2 = 0.261).

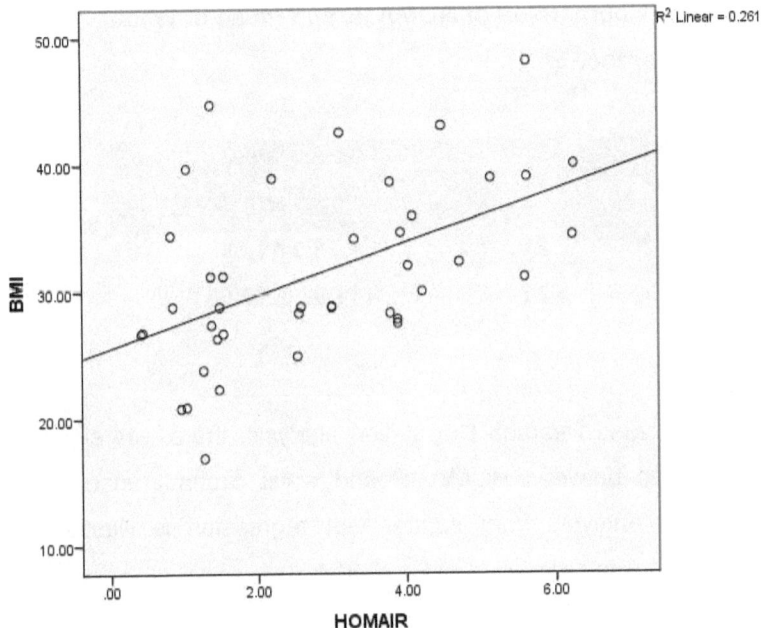

Figure 10: Correlation between BMI and HOMA IR

3.5 WAIST CIRCUMFERENCE AND INSULIN RESISTANCE

Our study population had a wide range of waist circumference between 67 and 144 centimeter with a mean of 104.69 ± 12.77 centimeter. Comparison between mean of waist circumference with insulin resistance were made using a t-test. Analysis revealed significant difference ($p<0.05$) as illustrated in Table 5.

Table 5: Comparison of HOMA IR and mean of Waist Circumference

HOMA IR	N	Mean Waist Circumference
≤ 2.99	21	98.38 ± 11.51
> 3	21	111.00 ± 10.88

p=0.001

Using 2-tailed Pearson Correlation analysis, there was significant correlation between HOMA IR and waist circumference (r=0.59 p<0.05). Analysis from scatter plot regression is illustrated in Figure 11 with correlation of R^2=0.354.

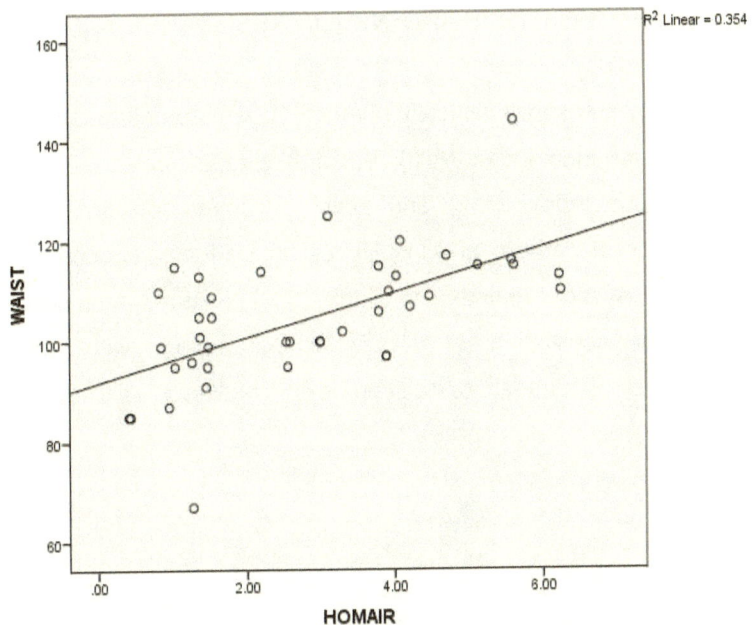

Figure 11: Correlation between waist circumference and HOMA IR

3.6 OSA PARAMETERS AND INSULIN RESISTANCE

This study measured clinically relevant OSA parameters including apnea hypopnea index (AHI), epworth sleepiness scale (ESS), Body Mass Index (BMI) and waist circumference (WC). The distribution of patients and insulin resistance for categorical OSA parameters are tabulated in Table 6. The table summarizes significant correlation of all these parameters with insulin resistance. Strongest correlation exist between AHI and IR (r=0.72).

Table 6: Distribution of patients across OSA parameters and HOMA IR values

Parameter	Category	Number of patients (n (%))		2-tailed Pearson Correlation (r value, p value)
		HOMA IR <=2.99	HOMA IR >3	
AHI	Normal	11 (26.2%)	3 (7.1%)	r= 0.72, p<0.05
	Mild	5 (11.9%)	2 (4.8%)	
	Moderate	3 (7.1%)	1 (2.4%)	
	Severe	2 (4.8%)	15 (35.7%)	
ESS	Normal	14 (33.3%)	3 (7.1%)	r= 0.47, p<0.05
	Mild	4 (9.5%)	7 (16.7%)	
	Moderate	3 (7.1%)	8 (19.0%)	
	Severe	0 (0%)	3 (7.1%)	
BMI	Underweight	1 (2.4%)	0 (0%)	r=0.51, p<0.05
	Normal	3 (7.1%)	0 (0%)	
	Preobese	6 (14.3%)	1 (2.4%)	
	Obese 1	8 (19.0%)	12 (28.6%)	
	Obese 2	1 (2.4%)	5 (11.9%)	
	Obese 3	2 (4.8%)	3 (7.1%)	

CHAPTER 4

DISCUSSION

This is the first study conducted in Malaysia looking at relationship of OSA and insulin resistance. It was a clinic-based sample in which patients were referred by general practitioners and physicians for overnight polysomnogram after presented with symptoms such as excessive daytime sleepiness, disturbed nocturnal sleep or insomnia. None of these patients were specifically referred for assessment of disorders of glucose metabolism associated with clinical signs of OSAS.

The findings of this study suggested that Obstructive Sleep Apnea (OSA) is significantly correlated to insulin resistance. Results demonstrated that subjects with OSA had a significantly greater HOMA-IR value ($p<0.05$). This result is further supported by a linear relationship seen on Pearson correlation study between AHI and HOMA-IR.

In many studies of insulin resistance related sleep disordered breathing, major confounding factor in the analysis is obesity. Measures of obesity include BMI, waist circumference and waist-hip circumference ratio. Earlier studies have demonstrated that obesity correlates significantly with insulin resistance. Ip *et al* in 2002 investigated the relationship between sleep disordered breathing and insulin resistance. They found out that obesity was the major determinant of insulin resistance but sleep-disordered breathing parameters (AHI and minimum oxygen saturation) were also independent determinants of insulin resistance.[4] In another study by Elmasry *et al* in 2001, they look at the association of diabetes mellitus and OSA in a sample of 116 age-stratified men with hypertension selected from subjects in a population-based study in Sweden. It was shown that although obesity was the main risk factor for diabetes mellitus, coexistent severe OSA may add to the risk independently.[25]

Insulin resistance in this present study was highly related to AHI, less with waist circumference and BMI. Analysis from scatter plot regression revealed a correlation result between HOMA IR and AHI of $R^2=0.529$. Therefore we concluded that the effects of AHI were greater than of obesity as correlation on scatter plot regression showed smaller value: BMI ($R^2=0.261$) and waist circumference ($R^2=0.354$). This result is comparable to more recent studies.

Punjabi *et al* in 2002 studied 150 healthy men to determine the metabolic consequences and community prevalence of sleep-disordered breathing. After adjusting for BMI and percent body fat, increasing AHI was associated with worsening insulin resistance independent of obesity.[9] There was also another paper by him in 2004 which investigated the association between severity of sleep-disordered breathing and insulin resistance by modeling the relation between AHI and HOMA index. It consisted of 2656 participants enrolled in the multicenter Sleep Heart Health Study. They too concluded that severity of AHI determined higher value of

HOMA index independently of BMI and waist circumference.[22] More recent study by Papanas *et al* in 2010 also concurred with our result, in which increased in serum glucose was significantly associated with OSA independent of BMI.[24]

Epworth Sleepiness Scale (ESS) was developed and validated by Dr Murray Johns. It is a simple, self-administered questionnaire which is widely used in quantifying the level of daytime sleepiness[1]. Nevertheless, ESS subjectively quantifies sleep propensity whilst the AHI is an objective value for the severity of OSA. A comparative audit of patient and partner scoring was carried out in Gloucestershire Royal Hospital. They found out that there was no mean difference between patient and partner perspective in ESS score ($P=.906$).[26] The partner perspective ($r=0.464$), but not the patient ESS ($r=0.305$) correlated with AHI. In their conclusion, ESS was found to be a poor predictor of AHI.[26] Their result was supported by another audit which tested upon Berlin Questionnaire and ESS as a screening instrument for OSA. ESS was found to have low to moderate sensitivity (45%) and specificity (81%), thus concluded ESS were of low value as screening tool.[27]

However, in this present study the mean ESS score was 11.36 (4.89) and a rise in ESS score was noted to be associated with an increase in the AHI index. The study also revealed significant association between mean of ESS and HOMA IR value ($p<.05$). There was also positive correlation seen between ESS and HOMA IR ($r=0.47$, $R^2=0.224$), although the effect was much smaller than

AHI and BMI. This was the first paper to assess the relation of ESS with insulin resistance especially in OSA patient.

Waist circumference is an independant prediction of relative disease risk and in the Asian population, it is a better indicator than BMI. [28] This is supported by many studies indicating significantly higher visceral adiposity in the East Asian population compared to Europeans at a given BMI.[29] In this study, waist circumference is used as opposed to waist hip ratio. Based on a prospective study of 48,287 patients by Seidell et al, it is shown that waist circumference alone could replace waist–hip ratio and BMI as a single risk factor for all-cause mortality and waist circumference is strongly predictive in young and middle-aged adults which is predominant in our study population.[30] Mean waist circumference in our study population was 104.69 cm. Up to our knowledge, there is no published data describing cut off points for waist circumference in East Asian population. This may be an area of potential future study owing to very high ethnic differences in distribution of waist circumference.

This study is important in the regional setting as the Southeast Asian population has different dietary practices and lifestyle compared to the Western counterpart where most papers on OSA and IR are reported. The Malaysian population has comparable nutrient intake with Singaporeans, Chinese and Japanese but consume proportionately more carbohydrates compared to British, Australian and New Zealanders.[31] The Malaysian population has slightly lower prevalence of IR compared to the British whereby findings of this study compliment the prevalence of IR in schizophrenic patients of 68%.[32]

In this study, we utilized ambulatory polysomnogram using a computer-assisted sleep study device (SOMNOCheck Effort Weinmann, Hamburg, Germany). This is a potential limitation as AHI may be under or over estimated. Future research could utilize the full, attended and manually scored polysomnogram to correct the imprecisions at the expense of a longer waiting time to perform the study as well as more tedious reporting efforts needed.

CHAPTER 5

CONCLUSION

In summary, the results of this study provide concrete evidence that Obstructive Sleep Apnea (OSA) is associated with insulin resistance and may have the following practical implications. Since insulin resistance is associated with type 2 Diabetes Mellitus and a risk for metabolic and cardiovascular complications, it appears useful for clinicians treating patients with diagnosed metabolic syndrome to bear in mind that they may have some reduction of sleep quality and that hyperglycemia increases the likelihood of OSA. Given that OSA itself aggravates insulin resistance, early specialist referral for diagnosis and management of this condition is beneficial. Further studies are needed to define the mechanism through which OSA promotes insulin resistance. We would also recommend further study to determine whether sustained treatment of OSA reverses the associated metabolic disturbance.

LIMITATION AND RECOMMENDATIONS

This study has a small sample size with one-year time frame, which is relatively not a good representation of subjects with or without OSA by potentially reducing statistical power. In order to determine a better correlation study, it will be appropriate to employ a larger scale of subjects with a match case-control design with BMI and matching demographic backgrounds.

In the evaluation of insulin resistance, the gold standard is the euglycemic clamp method. However it is expensive, invasive and labor intensive. Instead we use the HOMA IR which has been showed to be a useful guide to insulin resistance in normoglycemic individuals. It is simple and inexpensive alternative, used in large clinical and epidemiological study. Recent validation showed strong correlation between these two with correlation coefficient of -0.820.

The documentation of OSA was based on limited polysomnogram rather than the more appropriate full polysomnogram in-lab based. Finally, the lack of women subjects in this study, which influenced our ability to detect or find any relationship between insulin resistance and gender.

REFERENCES

1. Bassiri AG, Guilleminault C, Clinical features and evaluation of obstructive sleep apnea syndrome. In: Principals and Practice of Sleep Medicine. 3rd eds. Kryger MH, Roth T, Dement WC London: WB Saunders; 2000. p869-878.

2. Lee W, Nagubadi S, Kryger MH, Mokhlesi B. 2008. Epidemiology of obstructive sleep apnea: a population-based perspective. *Expert Rev Respir Med*; 2:349-364.

3. American Academy of Sleep Medicine. International Classification of Sleep Disorders. In: Diagnostic and Coding Manual. Second Edition. Westchester. 2005.

4. Ip MS, Lam B, Ng MM, Lam WK, Tsang KW, Lam KS. Obstructive sleep apnea is independently associated with insulin resistance. Am J Respir Crit Care Med. 2002; 165 (5): 670-676.

5. Young T, Palta M, Dempsey J, Skatrud J, Weber S, Badr S. The occurrence of sleep-disordered breathing among middle-age adults. N Engl J Med. 1993; 328: 1230-1235.

6. Koskenvuo M, Kaprio J, Telakiri T, Partinen M, Heikkila K, Saran S. Snoring as a risk

factor for ischaemic heart disease and stroke in men. Br Med J. 1987; 294: 16-19.

7. Tasali E, Mokhlesi B, Van Cauter E. Obstructive sleep apnea and type 2 diabetes: interacting epidemics. Chest. 2008; 133: 496-506.

8. Davies JJ, Turner R, Crosby J, Stradling JR. Plasma insulin and lipid levels in untreated obstructive sleep apnea: their comparison with matched controls and response to treatment. J Sleep Res. 1994; 3: 180-185.

9. Punjabi NM, Sorkin JD, Katzel LI, Goldberg AP, Schwartz AR, Smith PL. Sleep-disordered breathing and insulin resistance in middle-aged and overweight men. Am J Respir Crit Care Med. 2002; 165(5): 677-682.

10. Lobovitz HE. Insulin resistance: definition and consequences. Exp Clin Endocrinol Diabetes. 2001; 109(suppl 2): S135-S148.

11. American Diabetes Association. Consensus development conference on insulin resistance. Diabetic Care. 1998. 21: 310-317.

12. West SD, Nicoll DJ, Wallace TM, Matthews DR, Stradling JR. 2007. Effect of CPAP on insulin resistance and HbA1c in men with

obstructive sleep apnea and type 2 diabetes.*Thorax*; 62: 969-974.

13. Haffner SM, Miettinen H, Stern MP. The homeostasis model in the San Antonio Heart Study. Diabetes Care. 1997; 20: 1087-1092.

14. Laakso M. How good a marker is insulin level for insulin resistance?.Am J Epidemiol. 1993; 137: 959-965.

15. Otake K, Sasanabe R, Hasegawa R, Banno K, Hori R, Okura Y, Yamanouchi K, Shiomi T. Glucose intolerance in Japanese patients with obstructive sleep apnea. Inter Med. 2009; 48: 1863-1868.

16. Spiegel K, Knutson K, Leproult R, Tasali E, Van Cauter E. 2005. Sleep loss: a novel risk factor for insulin resistance and type 2 diabetes. *J ApplPhysiol;* 99: 2008-2019.

17. Stoohs RA, Facchini F, Guilleminault C. Insulin resistance and sleep-disordered breathing in healthy humans. Am J Res Crit Care Med. 1996; 154: 170-174.

18. Strohl KP, Novak RD, Singer W, Cahan C, Boehm KD, Denko CW, Hoffstem VS. Insulin levels, blood pressure and sleep apnea. Sleep. 1994; 17(7): 614-618.

19. Vgontzas AN, Papanicolaou DA, Bixler EO, Hopper K, Lotsikas A, Lin H, Kales A, Chrousos GP. Sleep apnea and daytime sleepiness and fatigue: relation to visceral obesity, insulin resistance and hypercytokinemia. J Clin Endocrinol Metab. 2000; 85: 1151-1158.

20. Al Delaimy WK, Manson JE, Willett WC, Stampfer MJ, Hu FB. Snoring as a risk factor for type II diabetes mellitus: a prospective study. Am J Epidemiol. 2002; 155(5): 387-393.

21. Meslier N, Gagnadoux F, Giraud P, Person C, Ouksel H, Urban T, Racineux JL. Impaired glucose-insulin metabolism in males with obstructive sleep apnea syndrome. Eur Respir J. 2003; 22 : 156-160.

22. Punjabi NM, Shahar E, Redline S, Gottlieb DJ, Givelber R, Resnick HE. Sleep disordered breathing, glucose intolerance, and insulin resistance: The sleep heart health study. Am J Epidemiol. 2004; 160: 521-530.

23. Coughlin SR, Mawdsley L, Mugarza JA, Calverley PMA, Wilding JPH. Obstructive sleep apnea is independently associated with an increased prevalence of metabolic

syndrome. European Heart Journal. 2004; 25: 735-741.

24. Papanas N, Steiropoulos P, Nena E, Tzouvelekis A, Skarlatos A, Konsta M, Vasdekis V, Maltezos E, Bourous D. Predictors of obstructive sleep apnnea in males with metabolic syndrome. Vascular health and risk management. 2010 ; 6: 281-286.

25. Elmasry A, Lindberg E, Berne C, Janson C, Gislason T, AwadTageldin M, Boman G. Sleep-disordered breathing and glucose metabolism in hypertensive men: a population based study. J Intern Med. 2001; 249: 153-161.

26. Hughes C. Can the Epworth Sleepiness Score predict Apnea-Hypopnea Index in Obstructive Sleep Apnea and hypopnea syndrome: A comparative audit of patient and partner scoring. ERS Annual Congress. 2011; Amsterdam.

27. Mensink A, Uil S, Kuipers B. Berlin questionnaire and Epworth sleepiness scale, useful screening instruments for obstructive sleep apnea syndrome? ERS Annual Congress. 2011; Amsterdam.

28. Klatsky AL, Armstrong MA. Cardiovascular risk factors among Asian Americans living in northern California. Am J Public Health. 1991;81:1423-1428

29. Kagawa M, Binns CB, Hills AP. Body composition and anthropometry in Japanese and Australian Caucasian males and Japanese females. Asia Pacific Journal of Clinical Nutrition, 2007; 16 Suppl 1:31-36

30. Seidell JC, Verschuren WM, van Leer EM et al. Overweight, underweight, and mortality. A prospective study of 48,287 men and women. Archives of Internal Medicine, 1996;156(9):958-963

31. Mirnalini K, Zalilah MS, Safiah MY, Tahir A, Siti Haslinda MD, Siti Rohana et al. Energy and Nutrient Intakes: Findings from the Malaysian Adult Nutrition Survey (MANS). Mal J Nutr. 2008; 14(1): 1-24.

32. Fairuz AR, Maniam T, Khalid BA. Prevalence of Insulin Resistance in Schizophrenia in HUKM. Med J Malaysia. 2007; Oct 62 (4): 290.3

APPENDICES

STUDY PROFORMA

Name:

Age:

Gender:

Race:

Marital status: married/single/divorce

History:

The Epworth Sleepiness Scale

0= would never doze

1= slight chance of dozing

2= moderate chance of dozing

3= high chance of dozing

SITUATION	CHANCE OF DOZING
Sitting and reading	
Watching television	
Sitting inactive in public place	
As a passenger in a car for an hour without a break	
Lying down in the afternoon when circumstances permits	
Sitting and talking to someone	
Sitting quietly after lunch without alcohol/ tea/ coffee	
In a car, while stopped for a few minutes in traffic	

The level of sleepiness are graded as follows:

    Normal : 0-9
    Mild   : 10-13
    Moderate: 14-19
    Severe : 20-23

Physical examination:

Height (cm)	
Weight (kg)	
Body mass index (BMI)	
Waist circumference (cm)	
Neck circumference (inch)	

Severity of sleep apnea on sleep study:

		SEVERITY
Number of AHI		
Lowest Oxygen saturation		

Insulin resistance:

Fasting insulin (µU/ml)	
Fasting glucose (mmol/L)	
Insulin resistance HOMA IR	

APNEA HYPOPNEA INDEX

Apnea Hypopnea Index	Severity
Less than 5 per hour	normal
5 – 15 per hour	mild
16 – 30 per hour	moderate
More than 30 per hour	severe

American Academy of Sleep Medicine 2005

BODY MASS INDEX

Underweight	<18.5
Normal	18.5 - <22.9
Preobese	22.9 - < 27.5
Obese 1	27.5 - < 35.0
Obese 2	35.0 - <40.0
Obese 3	> 40.0

Revision of BMI Cut-Offs in Singapore 2005

PATIENT INFORMATION SHEET

Study Title
Insulin Resistance In Patient With Obstructive Sleep Apnea: A Cross Sectional Study

Introduction
There are 2 types of sleep apnea: central and obstructive or mixed. Obstructive Sleep Apnea Syndrome (OSAS) is a more common morbid health problem. OSAS occurs when the air cannot flow into or out of the person's nose or mouth although effort to breath continues. OSAS patients may present with symptoms of daytime sleepiness, snoring and multiple episodes of choking or gasping during sleep. The polysomnography (PSG) is the gold standard for diagnosis of OSAS.

OSAS is a complex disorder and associated with multiple complications such as hyperinsulinemia, glucose intolerance, insulin resistance, central obesity and hypertension.

Insulin resistance refers to a reduction in the expected physiologic action of insulin. Increased insulin resistance is a primary characteristic of type 2 Diabetes Mellitus as well as an independent risk factor for hypertension and coronary heart disease.

What would the study involve?
In this study you will first undergo a polysomnography test to determine the diagnosis of OSAS, followed by venous blood sampling in the fasting state for the measurement of glucose and insulin to evaluate the value of insulin resistance.

The Benefits
Apart from the sleep study being done, thorough physical examination will tell us (researcher) and you with regards to your current health status. Participation in this study also will help to diagnose OSAS patient, to determine the prevalence of insulin resistance and to anticipate risk of developing type 2 Diabetes Mellitus.

The Risk

There are no additional risks involved, as the procedures involved in polysomnography test and blood sampling are part of the management of the patient.

Confidentiality

The result of the data obtained will be reported in a collected manner with no reference to a specific individual. Hence, the data from each individual will remain confidential. As a patient only you have the right to know the results of the analysis.

Do I have to take part?

The participation into this study is voluntary. If you prefer not to take part, you do not have to give reason and researcher will not be upset and your decision will not affect the treatment given. You may also withdraw at any point in time during the study.

Payment and compensation

You do not have to pay for participating in this study. Similarly, no payment is available to you for participating in this study. In the event that this study results in the development of any marketable product(s), you will have no ownership interest in the product and no right to share in any profits from its commercialization whatsoever.

If I have any questions, whom can I ask at any time point of the study?

Dr Siti Zulaili Zulkepli

Jabatan Otorinolaringologi

Pusat Perubatan UKM, 56000 Cheras

Tel : 03-91456057

CONSENT FORM

Title of project

Insulin Resistance In Patient With Obstructive Sleep Apnea: A Cross Sectional Study

Consent:

I have read the information on the research project stated above and I have also been given the explanation by medical officer about purpose of this document. I understand that I retained the absolute right over the tests and may withdraw at any time. I have also the right to know about the research conducted on me including information on the results of the research.

I,_____ (IC No:_____) agree/disagree to participate in this study.

I would like to know/don't want to know the result of this study

Signature : -----------------------

Date : -----------------------

Witness
Name :
IC :
Signature :
Date :

Medical Officer
Name :
IC :
Signature :
Date :

ACKNOWLEDGEMENT

The author(s) would like to acknowledge the financial contributions for this study which came from the Fundamental Research Grant of Universiti Kebangsaan Malaysia. We would like to express our gratitude towards the supporting staff of the Otorhinolaryngology Sleep Lab, Otorhinolaryngology Ward, Hospital Universiti Kebangsaan Malaysia for their efforts in supporting this study. Lastly, we would like to acknowledge the contributions by the Endocrinology team, Hospital Universiti Kebangsaan Malaysia, lead by Prof Dr. Nor Azmi bin Kamarudin for their timely contributions towards the study.

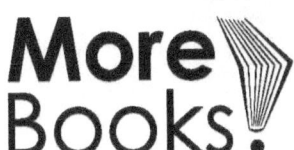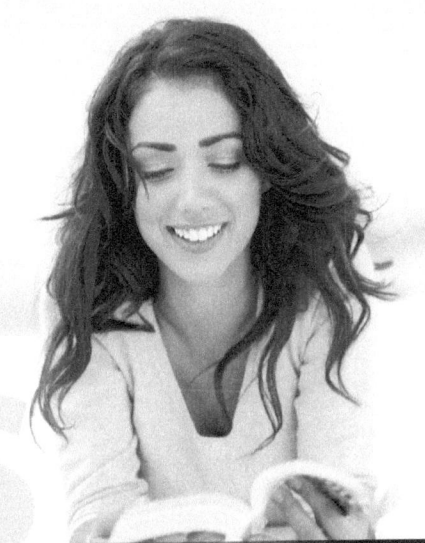

I want morebooks!

Buy your books fast and straightforward online - at one of the world's fastest growing online book stores! Environmentally sound due to Print-on-Demand technologies.

Buy your books online at
www.get-morebooks.com

Kaufen Sie Ihre Bücher schnell und unkompliziert online – auf einer der am schnellsten wachsenden Buchhandelsplattformen weltweit!
Dank Print-On-Demand umwelt- und ressourcenschonend produziert.

Bücher schneller online kaufen
www.morebooks.de

OmniScriptum Marketing DEU GmbH
Heinrich-Böcking-Str. 6-8
D - 66121 Saarbrücken
Telefax: +49 681 93 81 567-9

info@omniscriptum.com
www.omniscriptum.com

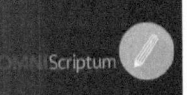

www.ingramcontent.com/pod-product-compliance
Lightning Source LLC
Chambersburg PA
CBHW031548210526
45464CB00003B/1213